THE DIET FOR SHEDDING BELLY FAT

IMPROVE YOUR LIFE BY CHANGING YOUR GUT

By

Amy W. White

THE DIET FOR SHEDDING BELLY FAT : IMPROVE YOUR LIFE BY CHANGING YOUR GUT

Before this document is duplicated or reproduced in any manner, the publisher's consent must be gained. Therefore, the contents within can neither be stored electronically, transferred, nor kept in a database. Neither in Part nor full can the document be copied, scanned, faxed, or retained without approval from the publisher or creator.

Table of contents

INTRODUCTION

Make time for yourself.

Chapter 4:

Develop steps quickly to fix gut harm.

Part II: Meals to feed your body
Here are some examples of gut-friendly meals:

Chapter 5:

Feed them the food they value the most.

Chapter 6:

Consume a lot of plant-based energy.

Chapter 7:

Remain true to consuming grains.

Six ways physical activity strengthens immunity

Body temperature rises with exercise.

Better sleep is a result of exercise.

Getting moving reduces inflammation.

Chapter 10: Supplemental probiotic use.

enhanced digestion and reduced signs of IBS and diarrhoea, among other digestive disorders.

Several well-liked probiotic supplements consist of:

INTRODUCTION

Your chances of losing weight and digesting food: Digestion is a complex process that involves breaking down the food you eat into smaller molecules that your body may utilise for energy and other purposes. Weight loss, on the other hand, is a bit more difficult. Nutrition, activity level, metabolism, and genetics are just a few of the factors that might influence your weight. To lose weight, you must create a calorie deficit by taking fewer calories than you burn. Weight loss and digestion are two closely related topics since the food you eat affects both your weight and your digestive health. What you eat impacts how your body digests and absorbs

nutrients, which affects how you feel and how your body operates.

To understand how weight reduction and digestion are connected, you must first understand digestive principles.

The process of breaking down the food you ingest into smaller molecules that may be absorbed by your body is the foundation of digestion. This method combines mechanical and chemical digestion. Mechanical digestion is the physical breaking down of food into smaller pieces that happens as you chew or when food passes through your stomach and intestines. The molecular breakdown of food molecules into even smaller molecules that your body can use is known as molecular digestion.

Enzymes, which are proteins that speed up chemical reactions, do this chemical digestion. Different enzymes degrade various types of substances, such as proteins, lipids, and carbohydrates.

PART 1.What exactly is going on with you? Food travels down your throat and into your stomach as you eat. Your stomach is a muscular organ that mixes food with digestive juices, which aids in further digestion. Gastric acid, often known as stomach acid, is the primary digesting liquid in your stomach. This acid is very acidic, with a pH of around 1-2. This acidity aids in the elimination of any potentially harmful microorganisms in the meal and also activates some of the enzymes that break down the food. As the food is mixed and broken down in the stomach, a sticky liquid known as chyme is produced.

The lower esophageal sphincter is the opening to your stomach. This ring-shaped muscle opens and closes the channel between your oesophagus and stomach as needed. The sphincter relaxes during digestion, allowing food to enter your stomach.

Muscles push food from the upper to the lower area of your stomach during digestion. The actual action begins at this point. Digestive juices and enzymes break down the food you chewed and swallowed here. It prepares it to provide energy to your body. Many digestive fluids and enzymes are produced by the stomach and mix with food. Following that, the stomach's strong muscles act like a blender to turn food into a usable form.

This procedure takes longer for certain foods than others. Carbohydrates, for example, degrade the fastest. This explains why many people recommend carb-heavy diets for a quick energy boost. Proteins need more time to digest and exit the stomach. Fats are the slowest of all. Water and other zero-calorie liquids empty the stomach the fastest.

When the stomach has finished its role in the digestive process, its contents are gently moved into a tiny tube at the stomach's base. This is known as the duodenum. It is the first stage of the small intestine. The next stage of digestion occurs here. Digestive fluids produced by organs such as the liver and pancreas help to keep the process of turning food into energy going.

Chapter 1

Introduction to Microbes:

Microbes are microscopic, unicellular animals that are invisible to the naked eye. Because they can only be seen under a microscope, they are sometimes known as microorganisms or microscopic beings. They account for nearly 60% of all living things on the planet.

The term "microbes" refers to a variety of unique life entities with varying sizes

and characteristics. Among these microbes are:

Bacteria

Fungi

Protists

Viruses

Archaea

Microbes may be both useful and harmful. Certain microbes cause significant infections and ailments, as well as the contamination of food and other items. Others, on the other hand, play an important part in maintaining environmental balance.

Let us examine the many types of microorganisms and their importance.

Microbes, often known as microorganisms, are tiny living creatures that are too small for the naked eye to see. Bacteria, archaea, fungus, and protists are among them. Bacteria and archaea are examples of single-celled microorganisms. Others, such as fungi and protists, may have many cells. Microbes play an important role in digestion. They live in your gut, also known as your gastrointestinal system, and aid in the digestion of meals. They also serve to maintain your gut healthy and protect you from potentially harmful bacteria.

Microbes are very important for a number of reasons. For starters, they aid in the digestion of our meals. Without

them, we would be unable to digest our meals and absorb the nutrients we need.

Second, they assist keep our gut healthy by keeping the right balance of bacteria and other pathogens. This protects us against diseases and infections. Third, they aid in the production of vitamins and other compounds that our bodies need. Finally, they assist our immune system function properly by teaching it to recognise and fight off hazardous infections and other illnesses.

Chapter 2:

Your overworked buddies:

When bacteria die, other microorganisms in our stomach break them down. This is known as microbial turnover. Microbial turnover is crucial because it contributes to the stability of the microbiome in our gut. Too much turnover may result in gut dysbiosis, which occurs when the equilibrium of microorganisms in our gut is upset. This may actually lead to a variety of health issues. Microbial overgrowth occurs when the bacteria in our gut are overworked. This may happen if we consume a high sugar, processed-food diet, which feeds the harmful bacteria in our gut. When this occurs, harmful bacteria might outweigh healthy bacteria, resulting in gut dysbiosis. This may lead to a variety of issues, including the ones I outlined above. But there is some good news! If you have signs of microbial overgrowth, Gut dysbiosis is a change in the balance of bacteria in our gut that may lead to a variety of health issues. These include gastrointestinal disorders such as IBS, inflammatory bowel disease, and even obesity. Gut dysbiosis has also been related to sadness, anxiety, and other mental health concerns in certain situations. There is also evidence that it may raise our risk of some cancers, such as colorectal cancer. All of this emphasises the importance of maintaining a healthy balance of bacteria in our gut! You can do things to restore the balance of bacteria in your gut.

Chapter 3:

Weight increase and microbiota balance:

You may foster a healthy balance of bacteria in your gut by doing a variety of things. To begin, it is critical to have a well-balanced diet rich in fruits, vegetables, and whole grains. These foods include prebiotics, which are compounds that feed the beneficial bacteria in our digestive tract. meals that may disrupt the healthy bacteria in our stomach, such as processed meals and sugary beverages, should also be avoided. In addition, getting adequate sleep and managing stress levels are vital since both may alter the balance of microorganisms in our stomach.

Digestive enzymes are proteins that aid in the breakdown of food into smaller molecules that our bodies can absorb. Our pancreas and small intestine create them, but they may also be present in some meals and supplements. Lipase, amylase, and protease are examples of digestive enzymes. Lipase aids in the digestion of lipids, amylase aids in the digestion of carbohydrates, and protease aids in the digestion of proteins. Taking digestive enzymes may help minimise microbial overgrowth symptoms including bloating, gas, and indigestion.

Make sure you eat your veggies.

Particularly the lush green ones! Vegetables are high in fibres, which are not digestible by humans but are absorbed by the healthy bacteria in your stomach. People that consume a diet high in fruits and vegetables are less prone to develop disease-causing germs. This are some wonderful examples of veggies that will help feed your microbes:

Leeks

Onions

Asparagus

Broccoli

Spinach

Artichokes

Sugar and processed meals should be avoided.

You're already too nice! Fast-digesting sugars, also known as monnosaccarides, are metabolised so swiftly that your bacteria never have a chance to eat them! If you consume too many simple carbohydrates on a daily basis, you risk actually starving your microbiota to death. Furthermore, hungry microorganisms will eat away at the lining of your colon, which may cause inflammation. To promote a happy and healthy microbiome, commit to change your diet to incorporate more foods containing complex carbohydrates.

Here's a list of sweet dishes that will satisfy both you and your stomach!

Honey

Chocolate, dark

Coconut Meal

Apples

Berries

Bananas

Mango

Yummy Sweet Potatoes

Also, watch out for the feared, hidden sources of monosaccharides. Sugar may find its way into meals that you wouldn't expect to find it in. Keep an eye on sugar levels in smoothies, nut butters, protein bars, salad dressings, and even yoghurt, a gut fave!

Probiotics are beneficial to your digestive system. Probiotics include live bacteria that will assist guarantee your stomach is inhabited by predominantly

beneficial germs. You can get a nice probiotic supplement at your local health food shop; however, ask your doctor which strains of cultures are best for you and the disease you're attempting to address. Many probiotic products claim to include living cultures but do not, so do your homework and consult with a qualified dietitian or health care professional before selecting a probiotic that is best for you.

Antibiotics should not be used.

Antibiotics are your gut's deadliest enemy if probiotics are its best buddy!

Antibiotics operate by killing all bacteria, making them incredibly useful for treating infections but very harmful to your microbiome. The antibiotic is unable to distinguish between healthy and dangerous gut microorganisms. They operate on the 'kill now, ask questions later' principle. Try to purchase antibiotic-free animal products, and if you must take an antibiotic, be sure to take a probiotic daily for the length of your prescription to help replace your gut flora.

Increase your consumption of prebiotic-rich foods.

Prebiotics nourish your microbiota! It is critical to feed these tiny guys in order to provide them with the energy they need to fulfil their critical role of controlling your enteric nervous system. Here is a list of dietary prebiotics that should be household staples:

Complete Grains

Apples

Leeks

Onions

Garlic

Extracts of cocoa

Garlic

Bananas

Asparagus

Nuts

Seeds

Extracted from red wine

Vegetables with Roots

Beans

Lentils

Chickpeas

Extracts from Green Tea

Go to the Gym

Your bacteria believe that if they are working hard to keep you healthy, you should work hard as well! Physically active persons have healthier and more diversified microbiomes. It also goes without saying that exercising is one of the finest ways to unwind after a hard day. Walking for 30 minutes a day may have a significant influence on your gut health and help these tiny microorganisms continue to ensure that your stress levels are regulated and your mental health is maintained.

Make time for yourself.

Say "no" more often and think about mindfulness, yoga, tai chi, or meditation. Creating a balanced lifestyle can benefit your gut and overall health, as well as your mental and emotional well-being. Stress may have a detrimental influence on your microbiome; hence, keeping a healthy microbiome is critical to

managing your stresses. If you are not cautious and do not allow yourself time to recuperate, you may find yourself in a vicious cycle.

Chapter 4:

Develop steps quickly to fix gut harm.

Have a meal rich in fiber. There are numerous reasons why fibre is important for gut health.

Consume a range of foods.

Eat fewer highly processed meals.

take in water.

Consume a food high in flavonoids.

Consume gently.

Consume fermented food.

Here's my quick guide to healing gut damage:

Start by removing the foods that are causing inflammation, like processed foods, refined carbs, and fake sweets.

Next, focus on adding nutrient-dense foods that are easy to stomach, like bone broth, fermented foods, and veggies.

Then, take vitamins that help improve gut health, like probiotics, L-glutamine, and zinc.

Finally, try to lower stress levels, as worry can hurt the gut lining.

These steps should help fix your gut and improve your general health!

 Step 1: Remove toxic foods from your diet. This includes prepared foods, refined carbs, and fake sweets.

Step 2: Replace these foods with nutrient-dense foods that are easy to stomach, like bone broth, veggies, and cultured foods.

Step 3: Rebalance your gut bacteria by taking probiotic pills or eating probiotic-rich foods, like kimchi, pickles, and kombucha.

Step 4: Restore your gut lining by taking vitamins like L-glutamine, zinc, and collagen.

Part II: Meals to feed your body

Food should be varied, bright, and high in fibre; however, remember that serving amounts should always be in the right proportions for your energy intake and should be eaten at regular times throughout the day, ideally three meals a day.

So here's our guide to the best foods for gut health: In no particular order, here are some tasty and odd things that are also good for your insides.

YOGHURT

Live yogurt is high in so-called beneficial bacteria, often known as probiotics. Look out for sugar-free, full-fat versions, and add your own food for a tasty breakfast. Yoghurt drinks can contain much numbers of bacteria that are good for the gut—far more than you would find in a normal yoghurt. Do be careful, though, as they can have a high sugar level.

KEFIR

This probiotic yoghurt drink is made by churning milk and is packed with good bacteria, which can help reduce a leaky ut. It developed in the hilly area between Asia and Europe, as well as Russia and Central Asia. It also makes a great addition to drinks and soups, or you can use it as a base for salad sauce (add lemon juice and spices).

MISO

Miso is made from fermented soy beans plus wheat or rice and includes a range of goodies, such as helpful bugs and enzymes. A spicy paste used in dips, sauces, and soup, it can also be used as a marinade for fish or tofu. It's a staple of Japanese food and ideal if you're avoiding dairy. There is doubt within the study that the bacteria successfully reach the gut; nevertheless, in areas where miso is a main fermented food source, the population has better gut health and less bowel illness.

SAUERKRAUT

This is freshly chopped cabbage that has been pickled. This great source of probiotics, fibre, and vitamins is best known as a German dish, but versions appear in Eastern and Central Europe. Choose a product that has not been pickled in vinegar, as that doesn't have the same benefits. It's delicious served with sausages and can be cheap and easy to make at home.

KIMCHI

This Korean treat of pickled veggies brings the benefits of probiotic bacteria along with vitamins and protein. Take it as a lively side dish with meat, salad, or eggs. It's so famous that Koreans say "kimchi" in the same way that we say "cheese" when they have their pictures taken.

SOURDOUGH

This is very popular at the time, but there's a good reason for that. Made by fermenting the dough, it's more edible than regular bread, and its energy drops slowly. It makes great toast, too.

ALMONDS

These have good bacterial qualities, which means they are a treat for your gut bugs. They are high in fibre and full of fatty acids and flavonoids. A handful of nuts makes an excellent snack when you're feeling peckish.

OLIVE OIL

Gut bacteria and gut germs like a diet of fatty acids and polyphenols. These are found in olive oil. Studies have shown that it helps lower gut inflammation. Use it for salad sauce or drizzle it over cooked veggies. Some studies have also found olive oil to be helpful in easing stomach problems and can also benefit your pancreas by lowering its requirement to make digestive enzymes.

KOMBUCHA

We all know water is important for gut health, but what else can you drink? Kombucha is a soured tea drink thought to have started in Manchuria that is full of healthy bacteria. It has a sharp, vinegary taste and can be used as a pleasant drink on its own or mixed with fruit and spices. It also makes the base for great drinks.

PEAS

Gut bugs need fibre to grow, so the more fruit and veggies you eat, the better. Peas are full of soluble and insoluble fibre to help keep your system intact. Also add peas to stir-fries, soups, or salads.

BRUSSELS SPROUTS

Much more than a holiday classic, they contain the kinds of fibre that good bacteria like and sulphur compounds that help fight bad bacteria such as H. pylori. Stir-fry with garlic and bacon for a beautiful side dish.

BANANAS

One of nature's handiest and best snacks, bananas are full of the kind of fibre that good bugs enjoy. They also contain healthy vitamins.

ROQUEFORT CHEESE

Live, messy, smelly French cheese* will give your gut bacteria a boost, but eat it in moderation. Add it to salads or spread it on your bread. While we cannot ensure that all of the bacteria survive digestion to be helpful, it is thought that other qualities help maintain some bacteria during digestion.

GARLIC

Garlic, with its antibiotic and antifungal effects, can help keep "bad" gut bacteria under control and help balance yeast in the gut. Use it as a flavouring for tasty recipes. The qualities of garlic work as a power source to allow the bacteria to do their job better, which overall improves gut health and can help heal your gut.

GINGER

Fresh ginger can help in the production of stomach acid, and it stimulates the digestive system to keep food going through the gut. Add fresh chopped ginger to soups, stews, shakes, or stir-fries. Pour hot water over chopped ginger to make refreshing ginger tea.

Here are some examples of gut-friendly meals:

Bone stock soup with veggies

Chicken, sweet potato, and broccoli

Salmon, veggies, and rice

Turkey, zucchini noodles, and avocado

Cauliflower crust pizza with veggies

Chickpea curry with rice

Zucchini lasagna

Greek yoghurt with berries and nuts

Eggs with greens and avocado

Grilled chicken salad with quinoa

All of these meals are packed with nutrients that will help feed your gut. Plus, they're easy to stomach and won't cause congestion.

Chapter 5:

Feed them the food they value the most.

Let's dig into the world of gut-friendly food. Ready?

To start, it's important to understand the idea of "food tribes". Food tribes are groups of foods that have similar traits, such as their impact on nutrition and gut health. The four main food tribes are:

Anti-inflammatory foods

Probiotic-rich meals

Prebiotic-rich foods

Fermented foods

Each food tribe serves a particular role in feeding the stomach. So, let's examine each tribe in greater depth.

Let's start with the anti-inflammatory food group. These are foods that help lessen inflammation in the stomach. Inflammation is a normal reaction of the defence system, but it may become extreme and cause problems. Anti-inflammatory foods may help quiet the immune system and improve digestive health. Some examples of anti-inflammatory foods are:

Turmeric

Ginger

Berries

Leafy greens

Extra-virgin olive oil

Nuts and seeds

Fish, particularly heavy fish like salmon and tuna

Herbs and spices like garlic, cinnamon, and thyme

Now, let's move on to the probiotic-rich food group. Probiotics are live bacteria that may boost the health of the gut microbiota. They may be found in fermented foods like:

Kefir

Yogurt

Sauerkraut

Kimchi

Kombucha

Tempeh

Miso

These meals may help improve the variety of the gut bacteria, which is important for general gut health. The gut microbiome is made up of billions of bacteria, and a varied microbiome is connected with improved health.

Prebiotics are kinds of food that support the good bacteria in the stomach. They're found in foods like:

Bananas

Apples

Onions

Garlic

Jerusalem artichokes

Asparagus

Legumes like beans and chickpeas

Barley

Whole grains

Dandelion greens

These meals help in promoting the growth of healthy germs in the stomach, which may improve digestion and lower the risk of certain sicknesses. We're on to the fermented food tribe. This tribe is a bit different from the other three tribes since it's made up of foods that have been pickled via a process called lacto-fermentation. This process produces lactic acid, which protects the food and gives it its unique sour taste. Some examples of fermented foods are:

Sauerkraut

Kimchi

Kefir

Miso

Tempeh

Kombucha

Pickles

Traditional sourdough bread

Yoghurt

These meals are not only tasty

Certain foods are high in good bacteria, called probiotics. They also include several vitamins and minerals that are needed for a healthy stomach. These include:

Vitamin B12

Vitamin K2

Folic acid

Calcium

Phosphorus

Iron

Potassium

Magnesium

Zinc

These nutrients are needed for a range of processes in the body, including blood cell growth, bone health, and energy creation. Additionally, fermented foods have been proven to improve the intake of other nutrients, such as vitamins.

If you prefer dairy products, you might consider moving from ordinary yoghurt to plain, sour yoghurt that includes active bacteria. This sort of milk is a great source of probiotics. You may also try adding a teaspoon of sauerkraut or kimchi to your lunch or supper. Sauerkraut is made from fermented cabbage, whereas kimchi is created from pickled veggies, including cabbage and radish. They both have a unique, somewhat sour taste that may add a wonderful bite to any meal.

Chapter 6:

Consume a lot of plant-based energy.

There are several possible benefits to eating plant-based proteins. First, plant-based protein is often lower in calories and fat than animal-based protein, which may be useful for weight reduction or weight control. Additionally, plant-based protein tends to be higher in fibre than animal-based protein, which may help improve fullness and control blood sugar levels. Plant-based protein sources also tend to include greater amounts of antioxidants, vitamins, and minerals than animal-based protein. Finally, some studies show that plant-based proteins may have positive effects on heart health and cholesterol levels.

There are a few possible downsides to counting totally on plant-based protein. First, plant-based protein sources may not offer all of the important amino acids that the body needs, which are usually found in animal-based protein sources. Additionally, certain plant-based protein sources, including beans, include chemicals called phytates, which might interfere with the absorption of key minerals like calcium and iron. Lastly, those with specific health problems, such as celiac disease or Crohn's disease, may find it difficult to receive sufficient protein from plant-based sources.

It's simple to receive plant-based sources of protein at the food store. Just look at all these options! These meals also tend to be rich in protein, vitamins, minerals, and other important nutrients.

- Beans

- Broccoli

- Chickpeas

- Greens

- Lentils

- Nut Butter

- Nuts and nuts

- Peas

- Potatoes

- Quinoa

- Seaweed

- Soy milk

- Spinach

- Tempeh

- Tofu

- Veggie Patties

Plant-based protein is protein that comes from plants, as compared to animals. Examples of plant-based protein include beans, peas, lentils, nuts, and seeds. Many whole grains, like quinoa and oats, are also great sources of plant-based protein. Plant-based protein may be a great option for people who are looking to reduce their diet of animal products or for those who are vegan or vegetarian. Plant-based protein is often lower in saturated fat and cholesterol and may be a good source of fibre and other minerals.

Plant-based protein refers to protein that is taken from plants rather than animals. Plant-based protein sources include legumes (such as beans, peas, and lentils), nuts and seeds, whole grains, and certain veggies. Unlike animal-based protein, plant-based protein does not include cholesterol or fatty fat. Additionally, plant-based protein sources tend to be lower in calories and higher in fibre than animal-based protein sources.

Chapter 7:

Remain true to consuming grains.

Grains are the edible seeds of plants that have been tamed for human use. There are two main kinds of grains: cereal grains and pseudocereals. Cereal grains include wheat, rice, maize, oats, barley, and rye. Pseudocereals, like quinoa and buckwheat, are officially not true grains but are usually eaten like grains and have similar nutritional values. Grains may be used to make bread, pasta, porridge, and other foods. They may also be crushed into flour for baking or used whole in meals like salads and soups.

Whole grains are ones that have been lightly treated, so they still include all three parts of the grain kernel: the bran, the germ, and the endosperm. The bran is the top layer of the grain, which is rich in protein and other nutrients. The germ is the core component of the grain, and it's rich in vitamins, minerals, and good fats. The endosperm is the middle part of the grain, which holds the majority of the grain's carbs and protein.

There is a big difference between grains and whole grains! As I mentioned, whole grains are barely treated, so they retain all three parts of the grain seed. On the other hand, most grains that are usually consumed are processed grains, which have been handled to remove the bran and germ. This makes them less healthy and less enjoyable. Some examples of polished grains include white flour, white rice, and de-germed cornmeal. So, it's crucial to seek out things branded as "whole grain" or "100% whole grain" to obtain the greatest nourishment from your grains.

Here's all you need to know about the benefits of grains.

Grains are a vital element of a healthy diet since they supply a range of nutrients, including carbs, fibre, and protein. Whole grains, such as wheat, brown rice, and quinoa, are especially healthy since they include more protein and nutrients than processed carbs. Eating whole grains has been linked to a number of health benefits, including a lower chance of heart disease, stroke, type 2 diabetes, and several forms of cancer.

Whole grains may also help you feel full and happy, which may assist with weight control. In addition, the fibre in whole grains may help lower cholesterol levels and improve gut health. And finally, whole grains include vitamins that may help protect against inflammation and cell damage. So there are many good reasons to make sure you're getting enough whole grains in your diet.

It might be tricky to make sure you're eating enough whole grains, but there are a few things you can do to make it easier. One easy method is to try to make at least half of the grains you eat whole. For example, if you usually eat cereal in the morning, try moving to a whole-grain kind. You may also seek out whole-grain choices like pasta, bread, and rice. Another piece of advice is to try different healthy grains, such as quinoa or farro, so you don't get tired of the same old choices. Finally, you may be sure to add whole foods into every meal.

Part III: Additional methods to improve the intestinal system

The intestinal tract, also known as the gastrointestinal tract, is a long tube that goes from the mouth to the anus. It's split into two main parts: the upper gastrointestinal tract and the lower gastrointestinal tract. The upper gastric system includes the mouth, oesophagus, and stomach. The lower gastrointestinal system includes the small intestine, large intestine, and rectum. The basic purpose of the gut system is to breakdown food and receive minerals. It also aids in the removal of waste from the body. The gut system is lined with millions of small finger-like structures called villi. The digestive system is also home to a great number of germs, which play a role in nutrition and general health.

When the gut system isn't healthy, it may lead to a variety of problems. One common problem is constipation, which may be caused by a lack of fiber, thirst, or a change in the normal muscle movements that carry food through the bowels. Diarrhoea is another common disease that may be caused by a variety of factors, including illness, food allergies, or irritable bowel syndrome. Other issues that might emerge when the digestive system isn't healthy include bloating, gas, and stomach pain. In certain cases, big problems like colon cancer or Crohn's disease might also appear.

There are a few things you can do to help fix your digestive system, but one of the most important is to focus on your food. Eating a high-fibre diet is important since fibre helps to add bulk to stool and keep things going through the bowels. Aim to eat at least 25 grammes of fibre per day from whole grains, fruits, veggies, and beans. Drinking enough water is also important since it helps keep things moving. Probiotics, or "good" bacteria, may also aid in improving the health of the gut system. You can receive probiotics from foods like milk and kefir.

Always try to keep your gut system healthy. First, it's crucial to eat a healthy, varied diet that includes lots of fruits, veggies, and whole foods. Getting adequate fibre is also crucial since it helps keep the digestive system moving. Drinking enough water is also important, as it helps to clean out toxins and keep the bowels moist. Regular exercise may also help keep a healthy digestive system by encouraging proper circulation and digestion. And lastly, controlling stress may also help to keep the intestine tract healthy since worry can upset the gut system.

Chapter 8:

Keep away from extra medicines.

An antibiotic is a sort of antibacterial drug useful against germs. It is the most important form of antibacterial drug for fighting bacterial illness, and antibiotic Medications are widely used in the avoidance and treatment of such illnesses. They may either kill or prevent the development of germs. A limited number of medicines also contain antiprotozoal effect. Antibiotics are not helpful against viruses such as the common cold or influenza. Medicines that control the growth of viruses are called antiviral medicines or antivirals rather than antibiotics. They are also not efficient against fungi; medications that reduce the growth of fungi include antifungal drugs. Antibiotics have been used since ancient times. Numerous cultures applied direct treatment of mouldy bread, with numerous references to its good qualities coming from ancient Egypt, Nubia,China,Serbia , Greece, and Rome. The first individual to clearly record the use of moulds to cure illnesses was John Parker (1567–1650). Antibiotics changed health in the 20th century. Alexander Fleming (1881–1955) developed present-day penicillin in 1928, whose broad usage proved immensely advantageous throughout warfare.

However, the effectiveness and cheap availability of antibiotics have also led to their misuse, and certain germs have developed tolerance to them. The World Health Organisation has classified antibiotic resistance as a global "serious threat [that] is no longer a prediction for the future; it has the potential to affect anyone, of any age, in any country, in any region of the world. Global death linked to antibiotic resistance hit 1.27 million in 2019.

Before the early 20th century, treatments for illnesses were based mostly on medical legends. Mixtures having antibacterial properties that were applied in treatments for diseases were described over 2,000 years ago. Many ancient societies, like the ancient Egyptians and ancient Greeks, employed specifically chosen mould and plant components to fix diseases. Nubian mummies examined in the 1990s were found to hold large amounts of tetracycline. The beer made during that time was conjectured to have been the cause.

The use of antibiotics in modern medicine started with the finding of manufactured antibiotics made from dyes. Various essential oils have been found to have antibacterial benefits. Along with this, the plants from which these oils have been gathered may be employed as specialist antibacterial agents.

Antibiotics are medicines that are used to treat bacterial infections. They work by killing the germs or stopping them from multiplying, which helps the body to fight off the sickness. There are many different sorts of antibiotics, and they're usually given based on the exact type of illness a person has. Some famous examples of antibiotics are penicillin, amoxicillin, and ciprofloxacin. It's vital to take antibiotics exactly as suggested by a doctor and to finish the whole course of therapy, even if symptoms lessen. Stopping medicines early might lead to a return of the illness.

Here are some of the main downsides of taking too many antibiotics:

• Antibiotic resistance, which may make illnesses harder to treat.

• Digestive problems include diarrhoea, sickness, and stomach pain.

• A weaker immune system makes it easier to become ill.

• Fungal illnesses, such as yeast infections and thrush.

• Allergic reactions include itching, swelling and rash.

• Other side effects, such as dizziness, headache, and tiredness.

So, it's vital to only take antibiotics when they're truly needed and to follow the advice for taking them exactly.

Here's some tips on how to avoid taking too many antibiotics:

• Only use medicines when suggested by a doctor.

• Always finish the whole course of medicines, even if you feel better.

• Talk to your doctor if you face any adverse effects.

• Ask your doctor whether antibiotics are actually necessary and consider alternative treatment choices.

• Take probiotics to help reset the balance of healthy bugs in your stomach.

• Follow healthy living habits, including eating a balanced diet and getting adequate sleep.

• Be aware of the signs of drug resistance and get treatment if you think you may have it.

Using too many medicines or using them for too long might have some dangerous consequences. For one, it may develop antibiotic resistance, which means that the germs grow immune to the drugs and no longer respond to treatment. This may make infections more difficult to fix and possibly lead to life-threatening illnesses. Additionally, overuse of antibiotics may cause the healthy bacteria in the stomach to be removed, leading to digestion problems and a weaker immune system.

Finally, it may also lead to fungal illnesses because the antibiotics might kill the helpful bacteria that help keep fungus growth under control.

Chapter 9:

Work out to strengthen your system.

Could building your immune system and preventing bacterial and viral infections be significantly aided by exercise?

It seems that staying healthy and preventing illnesses are aided by engaging in regular physical activity. This is due to the fact that exercise improves overall health, which may strengthen the operation of your immune system. This article discusses the idea that exercise might boost immunity and provides some guidance on whether it's still advisable to work out while you're sick. Increasing your body's immunity is only one of the many benefits that exercise provides. There is one important disclaimer, though: how often, how long, and how hard you exercise matters.

Studies indicate that moderate-intensity exercise is superior for boosting immunity. For the best benefits of exercise in strengthening the immune system, one should generally exercise for 60 minutes or less, at a moderate to high intensity. Your immune system and metabolism continue to develop if you do this on a regular or almost daily basis, building on the gains you have already made. Conversely, ongoing high-intensity exercise may weaken your immune system, especially if you don't get enough rest in between workouts.

Whether you are training for a marathon or other endurance event, or you are a competitive athlete, this is an important issue to address. In such cases, be very careful to give your body enough time to heal.

Prior to discussing how exercise might support your immune system, it's important to consider how much exercise you probably need for overall health.

The majority of people should engage in 150–300 minutes of moderate-intensity aerobic exercise or 75 minutes of

vigorous physical activity each week, according to the U.S. Department of Health and Human Services (HHS). Additionally, the HHS advises doing muscle-strengthening activities on at least two days a week that target all of the major muscle groups in your arms, shoulders, chest, belly, hips, legs, and back.

Getting moving on most days of the week is a great way to improve your overall health and wellbeing. If you want to work on boosting your immune system, this is also a great place to start.

Six ways physical activity strengthens immunity

Your body is shielded against infections, viruses, and other pathogens by a strong immune system.

These six activities may strengthen your immune system.

Exercise strengthens immunity inside cells. A 2019 research study found that by improving your body's immune cell circulation, moderate-intensity exercise may improve cellular immunity. By detecting it early on, this better prepares your body for a possible sickness.

Studies have shown that engaging in moderate-to-intense aerobic exercise for less than 60 minutes (on average, 30–45 minutes) improves the immune system's best defensive cells' recruitment and circulation. According to these findings, engaging in regular exercise may boost immune defence function by increasing infection resistance and improving your body's ability to fight off infectious agents that have already taken hold in your body.

Body temperature rises with exercise.

Your body temperature will increase throughout most forms of exercise, unless you're moving at a snail's speed, and it will remain high for a brief period of time thereafter.

Why does this matter? It's a widely accepted belief that this brief increase in body temperature that occurs during and after exercise may help your body fight off infections and better handle sickness, just as a fever does.

Nevertheless, it's critical to acknowledge that there is no empirical support for this theory.

This brief rise in temperature is not as harmful to your health as a fever, but it might still have some benefits for your immune system.

Better sleep is a result of exercise.

Frequent physical activity may enhance both the amount and quality of sleep overall. This is fantastic news since some immune system components may be negatively impacted by sleep deprivation. In adults with mild sleep loss, there may be a higher risk of infection as well as the emergence of metabolic and

cardiovascular issues due to a reduction in antibodies and the production of inflammatory cytokines.

Diabetes, heart disease, and other illnesses are reduced by exercise.

Exercise may lower resting heart rate, raise HDL (good) cholesterol, prevent or delay the onset of type 2 diabetes, and reduce cardiovascular risk factors.

If you have any of these conditions, your immune system may have a harder time fighting off infections and viral diseases like COVID-19.

Stress and other diseases, including depression, are reduced by exercise.

Exercise is valued by individuals for the reason that it reduces stress, especially after a demanding workday.

More specifically, moderate-intensity exercise may positively modify the brain's neurotransmitters that regulate mood and behaviour while decreasing the synthesis of stress hormones.

Exercise also helps you proactively handle stress with more resilience and a better mood, which may provide you a preventative edge against stress.

Certain research indicates that depressive and stressful conditions may significantly impact the immune system's ability to function normally, resulting in a low-grade chronic inflammation that fosters illnesses, infections, and other conditions.

Getting moving reduces inflammation.

Your body naturally employs inflammation as an immune system response to fight against infections or toxins. Not all inflammation is harmful at first, but if left uncontrolled, early reactions may develop into chronic inflammation, which can result in a variety of inflammatory illnesses. Exercise helps manage the immune response and reduce inflammation, according to research, but the intensity of the workout counts. Research indicates that although prolonged high-intensity exercise sessions may actually exacerbate inflammation, moderate-intensity exercise reduces inflammation. The key lesson? Your body's inflammatory immune response may be more effective when you exercise moderately and get enough rest, which lowers your chance of developing chronic inflammation.

Any physical activity that increases heart rate and gets your body moving is considered exercise. It offers several benefits for the body and the mind and is essential for overall health and wellbeing. Exercise comes in a variety of forms, ranging from strength training and flexibility routines like yoga and Pilates to cardiovascular sports like swimming and running. Exercise includes even everyday activities like walking and gardening. Finding something you like and incorporating it into your everyday routine is the goal. Exercise has many health benefits, including:

• Better health of the heart

.Decreased likelihood of long-term ailments.

• Improved mood and mental well-being.

• Higher vigour levels

Frequent exercise may help you feel better emotionally, sleep better, lower stress, and increase the flow of immune cells throughout your body—all of which are benefits of a strong immune system.

Chapter 10: Supplemental probiotic use.

Dietary supplements containing live bacteria or yeast are known as probiotics. These supplements include what are known as probiotics, which are bacteria or yeast that may help improve intestinal health. Probiotic supplements are available in a variety of forms, such as tablets, capsules, powders, and even foods like kefir and yoghurt. The most common probiotic strains found in supplements are Bifidobacterium and Lactobacillus. Probiotics are well recognised to provide a number of health benefits, such as: • enhancing digestion and reducing symptoms associated with digestive disorders.

• strengthening the immune system.

• Inflammation reduction

By reestablishing the proper balance of beneficial bacteria in the digestive system, probiotic supplements may improve gut health. The following are a few benefits of probiotic supplementation:

Enhanced digestion and reduced signs of IBS and diarrhoea, among other digestive disorders.

• a reduction in the frequency of respiratory illnesses.

• a decrease in eczema and other skin disease symptoms.

• Reduced stress and enhanced mental health

• Improved absorption of nutrients

• a greater ability to withstand the effects of antibiotics.

Selecting a probiotic supplement of superior quality that contains a wide range of bacterial species is essential.

Several well-liked probiotic supplements consist of:

One of the most widely used probiotics that can be found in supplements is Lactobacillus acidophilus, which is known to support immune system, skin, and digestive health.

Probiotic Bifidobacterium lactis is found in dairy products and is known to support immunological and digestive health.

The probiotic Lactobacillus rhamnosus is said to help with eczema, diarrhoea, and other skin conditions.

The probiotic Lactobacillus plantarum is meant to help with digestion.

Section IV: Attend to your stomach. Weight reduction meal plans, diets, and maintenance advice Losing weight and taking care of your stomach go hand in hand. To help you get on track, consider these suggestions:

Consume a diet high in fruits, vegetables, whole grains, and other fiber-rich foods.

Consume foods high in probiotics, such as kefir, sauerkraut, and yoghurt.

Eat less processed and sugar-filled meals.

To stay hydrated, take in a lot of water.

Ensure that you are receiving enough rest and exercise.

Lower your degree of stress.

See a physician or nutritionist if you need special assistance.

You'll find that attending to

The goal of the diet trials is to reduce visceral fat.

You must create a calorie deficit—that is, consume less calories than you expend—in order to lose weight. Aim for a 300–500 calorie daily deficit for a gradual and sustainable weight loss. You may do this by making simple changes like eating smaller portions, choosing

healthier snacks, and getting more exercise. Additionally, I'll recommend meals that are strong in protein and fibre to help you feel fuller for longer and avoid cravings.

Okay, that's great! I recommend starting your day with a high-protein, high-fiber breakfast, such as a veggie-packed melet or muesli with Greek yoghurt and berries. Choose a lunch that is high in vegetables and lean protein, such brown rice with beans and veggies or grilled chicken with a salad. Choose small handfuls of nuts or an apple with peanut butter as your snack. Choose a lean entrée such as chicken or fish, along with a side of vegetables and healthy carbs. In order to feel more energised and resist the need to overeat, it's also critical to obtain adequate sleep and drink enough of water.

It's important to understand, nevertheless, that losing weight in a specific area of the body is not possible with spot reduction. Not only in your belly, but throughout your whole body, you will lose weight. Nonetheless, you may reduce your overall body fat percentage and see a decrease in your belly fat by following a healthy diet and engaging in regular exercise. All you need to do is persevere and have patience, and you will start to see results!